Living with Coronary Artery Disease: Navigating the Journey to Heart Health

By

DR. KINGSLEY NEWMAN

This Book is Dedicated to my beloved son,
Richard.
You have been my rock through every chapter of
my life. Your birth has stood as a pillar of strength
and   inspiration   to   my   life.

TABLE OF CONTENT

Epilogue: Empowering Yourself for a

Heart-Healthy Future

This book aims to provide comprehensive insights, practical advice, and emotional support for individuals navigating life with coronary artery disease, fostering a holistic approach to heart health.

CHAPTER ONE:

UNDERSTANDING CORONARY

HEART DISEASE

Exploring the Basics: What is Coronary Artery Disease?

Coronary Artery Disease (CAD) lies at the heart of cardiovascular health concerns, affecting millions of individuals worldwide. To comprehend the intricacies of CAD, it is essential to delve into the fundamental aspects of this condition. At its core, CAD involves the gradual buildup of plaque within the coronary arteries, the blood vessels responsible for supplying oxygen and nutrients to the heart muscle.

The process begins with atherosclerosis, where fatty deposits, cholesterol, and other substances accumulate along the inner walls of the coronary arteries, forming plaques. Over time, these plaques may harden or rupture, leading to the development of blood clots that can partially or completely block blood flow to the heart. This restricted blood supply, known as ischemia, can result in chest pain (angina) or, in severe cases, trigger a heart attack (myocardial infarction).

Understanding the risk factors for CAD is crucial. Lifestyle factors such as poor diet, lack of physical activity, smoking, and excessive alcohol consumption contribute significantly. Additionally, genetic predispositions, age, and pre-existing conditions like diabetes and hypertension play roles in increasing susceptibility.

Regular check-ups, diagnostic tests, and collaboration with healthcare providers are vital for early detection and management of CAD. By comprehending the basics of CAD, individuals can take proactive steps toward prevention, adopt heart-healthy lifestyles, and navigate the challenges associated with this condition effectively.

Risk Factors: Identifying and Managing Your Risks

Identifying and managing risk factors is a pivotal aspect of proactively addressing coronary artery disease (CAD). Recognizing the various elements that contribute to the development or exacerbation of CAD empowers individuals to take control of their cardiovascular health.

1. Lifestyle Factors:
Unhealthy lifestyle choices significantly contribute to CAD. Poor dietary habits, characterized by high levels of saturated and trans fats, cholesterol, and sodium, play a substantial role. Sedentary behavior and lack of regular physical activity further escalate the risk. Smoking, a major risk factor, damages blood vessels and accelerates the progression of atherosclerosis.

2. Genetic Predisposition:
Understanding one's family medical history is crucial, as genetics can influence an individual's susceptibility to CAD. If close relatives have a history of heart disease, individuals may have a higher inherent risk. Genetic testing can provide insights into specific risk factors and guide personalized preventive measures.

3. Age and Gender:
Advancing age is a non-modifiable risk factor for CAD, with risk increasing significantly after the age of 45 for men and 55 for women. Men generally face a higher risk earlier in life, while post-menopausal women catch up in risk due to hormonal changes.

4. Medical Conditions:
Certain health conditions, such as diabetes, hypertension, and obesity, amplify the risk of CAD. Effective management of these conditions through medication, lifestyle adjustments, and regular medical check-ups is crucial in mitigating CAD risk.

5. Stress and Mental Health:
Chronic stress and untreated mental health issues contribute to CAD. Stress management techniques, mindfulness practices, and seeking mental health support are integral components of risk reduction.

Managing Your Risks:
Taking charge of one's health involves making conscious lifestyle changes. Adopting a heart-healthy diet, engaging in regular physical activity, and quitting smoking are paramount. Regular health check-ups and screenings enable early detection and intervention. Collaborating closely with healthcare providers to manage conditions

like diabetes and hypertension ensures comprehensive risk management.

Empowering individuals to identify and address these risk factors equips them with the tools needed for effective CAD prevention and management, fostering a proactive approach to heart health.

The Role Of Genetics In Coronary Artery Disease

The role of genetics in coronary artery disease (CAD) is a complex interplay between inherited factors and the influence of an individual's genetic makeup on cardiovascular health. Understanding how genetics contribute to CAD is crucial for developing personalized prevention and treatment strategies.

1. Genetic Predisposition:
Genetic factors significantly contribute to an individual's predisposition to CAD. If there is a family history of heart disease, especially if it involves close relatives such as parents or siblings, the risk of CAD may be higher. Specific gene

variants can influence cholesterol metabolism, blood clotting, and the development of atherosclerosis, impacting the overall risk profile.

2. Polygenic Risk Scores:
Advancements in genetic research have led to the development of polygenic risk scores (PRS) that assess an individual's genetic susceptibility to CAD based on multiple genetic markers. These scores provide a more comprehensive understanding of the genetic component, allowing for more targeted interventions and monitoring.

3. Single Nucleotide Polymorphisms (SNPs):
Researchers have identified specific genetic variations, known as single nucleotide polymorphisms (SNPs), associated with an increased risk of CAD. These variations can affect various biological processes, including inflammation, lipid metabolism, and blood vessel function.

4. Gene-Environment Interactions:
While genetics plays a significant role, it interacts with environmental factors. Unhealthy lifestyle choices, such as a poor diet or lack of physical activity, can amplify the impact of genetic predisposition. Conversely, adopting a heart-healthy lifestyle can mitigate genetic risks and promote cardiovascular well-being.

5. Inherited Conditions:
Certain genetic conditions, such as familial hypercholesterolemia, directly impact cholesterol levels and significantly increase the risk of CAD. Recognizing and managing these conditions through genetic testing and targeted interventions are essential for effective prevention.

Integrating Genetic Information into Healthcare:
The integration of genetic information into routine healthcare practices allows for more personalized risk assessments. Genetic counseling and testing can provide individuals with valuable insights into their inherited risk, enabling them to make informed decisions about lifestyle modifications, screenings, and preventive measures.

In conclusion, the role of genetics in CAD underscores the importance of a personalized and comprehensive approach to cardiovascular health. By understanding genetic predispositions and leveraging advancements in genetic research, individuals and healthcare providers can collaboratively work toward tailored strategies for CAD prevention and management.

CHAPTER TWO: Diagnosis and Medical Insights

Diagnostic Tests: From Angiograms to Stress Tests

Diagnostic tests play a crucial role in the comprehensive evaluation and management of coronary artery disease (CAD). From angiograms to stress tests, these procedures provide valuable insights into the condition of the heart, guiding healthcare professionals in making informed decisions about treatment and prevention.

1. Angiograms:
Angiography is a primary diagnostic tool for CAD. Coronary angiograms involve injecting a contrast dye into the coronary arteries and capturing X-ray images. This allows healthcare providers to visualize any blockages or abnormalities in the blood vessels supplying the heart. Angiograms are

instrumental in determining the extent and severity of coronary artery blockages.

2. Electrocardiogram (ECG or EKG):
Electrocardiograms record the electrical activity of the heart and are commonly used for CAD assessment. Changes in the ECG pattern can indicate insufficient blood flow to the heart muscle. Continuous monitoring or stress testing with ECG helps identify abnormalities that may not be evident during rest.

3. Stress Tests:
Stress tests, such as exercise stress tests or pharmacological stress tests, assess how the heart responds to an increased workload. These tests help detect CAD-related abnormalities that may not be apparent at rest. Stress tests are particularly valuable in evaluating symptoms like chest pain, assessing exercise capacity, and determining the effectiveness of ongoing treatment.

4. CT Angiography:
Computed Tomography (CT) angiography provides detailed images of the coronary arteries without the need for invasive procedures. It uses X-rays and computer technology to create cross-sectional images of the heart, helping identify plaque buildup, blockages, and other abnormalities.

5. Nuclear Stress Testing:
This specialized stress test involves injecting a small amount of radioactive material into the bloodstream. Imaging equipment detects the radioactive substance, highlighting areas of the heart with reduced blood flow. Nuclear stress testing provides valuable information about coronary blood flow and helps assess the overall functioning of the heart.

6. Blood Tests:
Blood tests, such as lipid profiles and cardiac biomarker assays, are essential for CAD diagnosis and monitoring. Elevated cholesterol levels and the presence of specific biomarkers like troponin can indicate heart muscle damage, aiding in the identification of a heart attack or ongoing cardiac stress.

7. Coronary Calcium Scoring:
This non-invasive imaging technique measures the amount of calcium in the coronary arteries, indicating atherosclerotic plaque buildup. Coronary calcium scoring assists in risk stratification and helps healthcare providers determine the appropriate course of action.

Incorporating these diagnostic tests into CAD evaluation enables a comprehensive understanding of the patient's cardiovascular health. By combining imaging, stress assessments, and laboratory results, healthcare professionals can tailor treatment plans, monitor disease progression, and empower individuals to actively participate in their heart health journey.

Collaborating with Healthcare Providers

Collaborating with healthcare providers is a cornerstone of effective coronary artery disease (CAD) management, fostering a partnership between individuals and their healthcare teams. This collaboration is instrumental in ensuring a holistic approach to heart health and personalized care.

1. Establishing Open Communication:
Effective collaboration begins with open and transparent communication between individuals and healthcare providers. Sharing detailed medical histories, lifestyle choices, and any concerns or symptoms allows for a comprehensive understanding of the individual's health status.

2. Regular Check-ups and Monitoring:
Scheduled check-ups and monitoring are essential components of CAD management. Regular visits

to healthcare providers enable the timely assessment of risk factors, medication adjustments, and the evaluation of the overall effectiveness of the treatment plan. This proactive approach helps catch potential issues early and prevents complications.

3. Shared Decision-Making:
Collaboration involves shared decision-making, where individuals actively participate in the choices regarding their healthcare. Healthcare providers offer guidance based on medical expertise, while individuals contribute insights into their preferences, values, and lifestyle considerations. This collaborative decision-making empowers individuals to take ownership of their health.

4. Treatment Plan Customization:
Healthcare providers tailor treatment plans based on the unique needs of each individual. Factors such as age, coexisting medical conditions, genetic predispositions, and lifestyle choices are taken into account when developing interventions. This personalized approach enhances treatment effectiveness and encourages adherence.

5. Lifestyle Counseling:
Collaboration extends to lifestyle modifications, which are fundamental in CAD management. Healthcare providers play a pivotal role in offering

guidance on adopting heart-healthy behaviors, including dietary changes, regular exercise, smoking cessation, and stress management. Collaborative goal-setting ensures that lifestyle changes are realistic and sustainable.

6. Medication Management:
Individuals collaborate with healthcare providers to manage medications effectively. Understanding the purpose, potential side effects and proper administration of medications is crucial. Regular medication reviews allow for adjustments as needed to optimize CAD control while minimizing adverse effects.

7. Educating and Empowering Individuals:
Healthcare providers serve as educators, providing individuals with the knowledge and tools needed to make informed decisions about their heart health. Educational sessions cover topics such as understanding CAD, recognizing symptoms, and the importance of preventive measures. Empowered individuals are better equipped to actively engage in their care.

8. Emotional Support and Well-being:
Recognizing the emotional impact of CAD, healthcare providers offer support and resources to address mental health needs. Collaborative discussions about stress, anxiety, and coping mechanisms contribute to overall well-being and

enhance the individual's ability to manage the emotional aspects of living with CAD.

In conclusion, a collaborative approach between individuals and healthcare providers forms the foundation for successful CAD management. By fostering open communication, shared decision-making, and personalized interventions, this collaborative partnership promotes optimal heart health and a higher quality of life for individuals affected by CAD.

Medications and Their Impact on CAD

Medications play a crucial role in the management and treatment of coronary artery disease (CAD), addressing symptoms, slowing disease progression, and reducing the risk of complications. Understanding the various medications and their impact is key to optimizing CAD control and promoting cardiovascular health.

1. Antiplatelet Medications:
Antiplatelet drugs, such as aspirin and clopidogrel, are commonly prescribed to prevent blood clot formation. By inhibiting platelet aggregation, these medications reduce the risk of clot-related events,

particularly in individuals with a history of heart attack or those who have undergone certain interventions like stent placement.

2. Statins:
Statins are lipid-lowering medications that play a central role in managing cholesterol levels. By inhibiting the production of cholesterol in the liver, statins help lower LDL (low-density lipoprotein) cholesterol and decrease the overall risk of atherosclerosis and coronary events.

3. Beta-Blockers:
Beta-blockers, such as metoprolol and carvedilol, are prescribed to manage blood pressure and reduce the workload on the heart. These medications can also help control irregular heartbeats (arrhythmias) and are beneficial for individuals with a history of heart failure.

4. ACE Inhibitors and ARBs:
Angiotensin-converting enzyme (ACE) inhibitors and angiotensin II receptor blockers (ARBs) are medications that help relax blood vessels, reducing blood pressure and lessening the strain on the heart. They are often prescribed to individuals with CAD, especially those with concurrent conditions like hypertension or heart failure.

5. Nitroglycerin:

Nitroglycerin is a vasodilator that helps widen blood vessels, improving blood flow and relieving angina symptoms. It is commonly used as a short-acting medication to alleviate chest pain and discomfort associated with CAD.

6. Calcium Channel Blockers:
Calcium channel blockers, such as amlodipine and diltiazem, are prescribed to relax blood vessels and reduce the heart's workload. These medications are often used to manage angina symptoms and control blood pressure in individuals with CAD.

7. Antiarrhythmic Medications:
For those experiencing irregular heart rhythms associated with CAD, antiarrhythmic medications may be prescribed. These drugs help regulate the heart's electrical activity, reducing the likelihood of arrhythmias.

8. Diuretics:
Diuretics, or water pills, may be prescribed to manage fluid retention and reduce blood pressure. This can be especially beneficial for individuals with heart failure, a condition that can be associated with CAD.

9. Lifestyle Medications:
In addition to traditional medications, lifestyle medications such as medications for smoking cessation or weight management may be

recommended to address specific risk factors contributing to CAD.

Monitoring and Adherence:
Regular monitoring by healthcare providers is essential to assess the effectiveness of medications and make adjustments as needed. Adherence to prescribed medications is crucial for optimal CAD management. Healthcare providers work collaboratively with individuals to address any concerns, manage side effects, and ensure that the medication plan aligns with overall health goals.

In conclusion, medications for CAD are diverse and serve specific purposes in managing the condition. Their impact extends beyond symptom relief, influencing risk factors and contributing to long-term cardiovascular health. Collaborative discussions between individuals and healthcare providers are essential to tailor medication plans to individual needs, and optimizing CAD management.

Chapter 3: Lifestyle

Modifications for Heart Health

The Power of a Heart-Healthy Diet

The power of a heart-healthy diet extends far beyond mere sustenance; it is a cornerstone in the prevention and management of coronary artery disease (CAD). A heart-healthy diet is not just a temporary regimen but a lifestyle that nurtures cardiovascular well-being, reducing the risk of heart disease and fostering overall health.

Central to this dietary approach is the emphasis on consuming nutrient-dense, whole foods. Fresh fruits and vegetables, whole grains, lean proteins, and heart-healthy fats become integral components. These foods provide a rich array of vitamins, minerals, antioxidants, and fiber, each playing a unique role in supporting heart health.

Crucially, a heart-healthy diet is synonymous with a reduced intake of saturated and trans fats, cholesterol, and sodium. By limiting processed and high-sugar foods, individuals can manage cholesterol levels and blood pressure, key risk factors for CAD. The incorporation of omega-3 fatty acids, found in fatty fish like salmon and flaxseeds, further contributes to cardiovascular health by reducing inflammation and promoting optimal heart function.

Equally significant is the impact of a heart-healthy diet on weight management. Maintaining a healthy weight is paramount for reducing strain on the heart and preventing the development or progression of CAD. By promoting weight loss when necessary and preventing obesity-related complications, a heart-healthy diet becomes a fundamental tool in the broader spectrum of cardiovascular care.

In essence, the power of a heart-healthy diet lies in its holistic influence on multiple facets of cardiovascular health. It is a proactive and empowering approach, empowering individuals to take charge of their well-being through the choices they make at every meal. Beyond preventing CAD, a heart-healthy diet nurtures vitality, energy, and a sustained sense of overall wellness.

Exercise and Physical Activity Guidelines

Exercise and physical activity are integral components of a heart-healthy lifestyle, playing a pivotal role in preventing and managing coronary artery disease (CAD). Comprehensive guidelines exist to help individuals incorporate effective and safe exercise routines into their daily lives, promoting cardiovascular health.

1. Aerobic Exercise:
Aerobic or cardiovascular exercise is a cornerstone of CAD prevention. These activities, such as brisk walking, running, cycling, and swimming, elevate the heart rate and improve circulation. The American Heart Association recommends at least 150 minutes of moderate-intensity aerobic exercise or 75 minutes of vigorous-intensity exercise per week for adults.

2. Strength Training:
Incorporating strength training exercises is crucial for overall fitness and heart health. This includes activities such as weightlifting or resistance training. Strength training enhances muscle mass, and metabolism, and helps control weight, all contributing to a healthier cardiovascular system.

3. Flexibility and Stretching:

Flexibility exercises, including stretching and yoga, improve joint mobility and reduce the risk of injuries. These activities also contribute to overall well-being, promoting relaxation and stress reduction. The American College of Sports Medicine suggests incorporating flexibility exercises 2-3 days per week.

4. Balance and Stability Training:
For older adults, balance and stability training are essential. Activities like tai chi or specific balance exercises can help prevent falls and injuries, ensuring a safe and sustainable approach to physical activity.

5. Gradual Progression:
It's crucial to start slowly and gradually increase the intensity and duration of exercise, especially for individuals who have been sedentary or those with pre-existing health conditions. This gradual progression minimizes the risk of injury and allows the body to adapt to increased physical demands.

6. Individualized Approach:
Exercise recommendations should be tailored to individual capabilities, preferences, and health status. Consulting with healthcare providers or fitness professionals ensures that the exercise routine aligns with specific health goals and considers any underlying medical conditions.

7. Consistency is Key:
Consistency is fundamental to reaping the benefits of exercise. Regular physical activity maintains cardiovascular fitness, helps control weight, and contributes to overall well-being. Finding enjoyable activities and establishing a consistent routine increases the likelihood of long-term adherence.

8. Listen to Your Body:
Individuals should pay attention to their bodies and modify exercise routines as needed. If there are signs of discomfort, pain, or other symptoms, it's essential to consult with healthcare providers promptly. Safety is paramount in any exercise program.

Adhering to these guidelines empowers individuals to take an active role in their cardiovascular health. Regular exercise not only reduces the risk of CAD but also contributes to improved mood, better sleep, and enhanced overall quality of life. It's a holistic approach that combines the strength of physical activity with the resilience of the human heart.

Stress Management and Mental Well-being

Stress management and mental well-being are integral aspects of a holistic approach to coronary artery disease (CAD) prevention and management. The intricate connection between mental health and heart health underscores the importance of adopting strategies to cope with stress and prioritize overall well-being.

1. Stress and Cardiovascular Health:
Chronic stress can contribute to the development and progression of CAD. The body's response to stress involves the release of hormones like cortisol and adrenaline, which, when prolonged, may lead to elevated blood pressure, inflammation, and an increased risk of atherosclerosis. Managing stress is, therefore, a crucial component of maintaining cardiovascular health.

2. Mindfulness and Relaxation Techniques:
Mindfulness practices, including meditation and deep-breathing exercises, are powerful tools for stress reduction. These techniques promote relaxation, lower blood pressure, and mitigate the impact of chronic stress on the heart. Incorporating

mindfulness into daily routines contributes to mental well-being and fosters a sense of calm.

3. Physical Activity as Stress Relief:
Regular physical activity not only benefits cardiovascular health but also serves as an effective stress-relief mechanism. Exercise triggers the release of endorphins, the body's natural mood elevators, helping combat stress and enhance overall mental well-being.

4. Adequate Sleep:
Quality sleep is essential for mental health and overall resilience against stress. Lack of sleep can contribute to increased stress levels and negatively impact cardiovascular health. Establishing consistent sleep patterns and creating a sleep-conducive environment is vital for stress management.

5. Social Connections:
Maintaining strong social connections and a support system is crucial for mental well-being. Social interactions, whether in person or virtually, provide emotional support and outlets for sharing concerns, reducing feelings of isolation and stress.

6. Time Management and Prioritization:
Effective time management and setting realistic priorities are essential for stress reduction. Individuals can benefit from organizing tasks,

breaking them into manageable components, and recognizing when to seek assistance or delegate responsibilities.

7. Seeking Professional Support:
When stress becomes overwhelming, seeking professional support through counseling or therapy can be beneficial. Mental health professionals can provide coping strategies, tools for managing stress, and a supportive environment for individuals navigating the challenges of living with or preventing CAD.

8. Holistic Approaches:
Holistic approaches, such as integrative therapies and alternative practices like acupuncture or biofeedback, can complement traditional stress management strategies. These approaches recognize the interconnectedness of mental, emotional, and physical well-being.

By addressing stress and promoting mental well-being, individuals can enhance their resilience against the impact of CAD. A comprehensive approach that integrates stress management into heart-healthy lifestyles not only supports cardiovascular health but also contributes to a more fulfilling and balanced life.

Chapter 4: Building a Support System

Navigating Relationships with Family and Friends

Navigating relationships with family and friends is a vital component of the intricate web that makes up an individual's journey with coronary artery disease (CAD). The diagnosis of CAD not only impacts the person directly affected but also reverberates through their social circles. Nurturing supportive and understanding relationships becomes paramount in managing the challenges and fostering overall well-being.

1. Open Communication:
Effective communication is the bedrock of navigating relationships amidst CAD. Sharing the diagnosis, treatment plan, and any lifestyle modifications with family and friends fosters transparency. This open dialogue creates a

foundation for mutual understanding and encourages empathy.

2. Education and Awareness:
Educating family and friends about CAD is crucial. Providing information about the condition, its management, and lifestyle changes helps dispel misconceptions and equips loved ones with the knowledge to offer meaningful support. Workshops or informational sessions may be beneficial in this regard.

3. Emotional Support:
CAD can evoke a range of emotions, from fear and anxiety to frustration. Creating an environment where individuals feel comfortable expressing their feelings without judgment is vital. Family and friends who offer a listening ear, emotional support, and encouragement play a pivotal role in alleviating the emotional burden associated with CAD.

4. Involvement in Care:
The inclusion of family members and friends in the care process can strengthen bonds and empower individuals with CAD. Attending medical appointments, participating in discussions about treatment plans, and collaborating on lifestyle modifications create a sense of shared responsibility and unity in facing the challenges of CAD.

5. Lifestyle Modifications as a Family Unit:
Adopting heart-healthy lifestyle changes is often
more successful when embraced collectively.
Engaging in activities like cooking heart-healthy
meals together, incorporating regular exercise into
family routines, and promoting a smoke-free
environment create a supportive ecosystem for
everyone's well-being.

6. Patience and Understanding:
Living with CAD may necessitate adjustments in
daily life. Patience and understanding from family
and friends during these transitions are invaluable.
Recognizing the individual's needs, respecting
their pace of adaptation, and offering
encouragement contribute to a positive and
supportive atmosphere.

7. Addressing Caregiver Stress:
For family members taking on caregiving roles, it's
essential to acknowledge and manage caregiver
stress. Balancing the responsibilities of caregiving
with self-care is crucial for both the caregiver's
well-being and the overall harmony of
relationships within the family.

8. Social Support Networks:
Encouraging the individual with CAD to connect
with support groups or engage in social networks
with others facing similar challenges can provide

an additional layer of emotional support. Sharing experiences with peers who understand the intricacies of living with CAD can be immensely beneficial.

9. Celebrating Milestones and Victories: Recognizing and celebrating milestones in CAD management, whether big or small, fosters a positive atmosphere. It reinforces the collective effort and resilience within the family and friend circle, motivating continued commitment to heart health.

Navigating relationships with family and friends in the context of CAD is a dynamic and evolving process. It requires continuous communication, adaptability, and a shared commitment to well-being. By fostering a supportive and understanding environment, individuals with CAD can navigate the challenges with resilience, knowing they have a network of loved ones standing beside them on their journey.

Joining Support Groups and Communities

Joining support groups and communities is a powerful strategy for individuals navigating the challenges of coronary artery disease (CAD).

These groups offer a unique and invaluable network where individuals can find understanding, shared experiences, and a sense of community, contributing significantly to their overall well-being.

1. Shared Understanding and Empathy:
Support groups provide a space where individuals with CAD can connect with others facing similar challenges. This shared understanding fosters empathy and creates a supportive environment where members can express their concerns, fears, and triumphs without judgment.

2. Information and Resources:
Being part of a support group allows individuals to access a wealth of information and resources related to CAD. Members often share insights into coping strategies, the latest medical advancements, and practical tips for managing the condition, contributing to a more informed and empowered community.

3. Emotional Support:
CAD can take an emotional toll, and support groups offer a platform for individuals to share their emotional experiences. Expressing feelings of anxiety, frustration, or even hope can be therapeutic, and the emotional support received from others who truly understand can be profoundly reassuring.

4. Practical Advice for Lifestyle Changes:
Managing lifestyle changes is a significant aspect
of living with CAD. Support groups provide a
space for members to exchange practical advice on
adopting heart-healthy habits, incorporating
exercise into daily routines, and making dietary
adjustments. This shared wisdom facilitates a
collective journey towards better heart health.

5. Motivation and Inspiration:
Witnessing the successes and resilience of others
within the support group can be motivating and
inspiring. Members share their triumphs over
challenges, fostering a sense of hope and
determination. This collective spirit encourages
individuals to stay committed to their CAD
management plans.

6. Caregiver Support:
Support groups are not limited to individuals with
CAD; they often include caregivers who play
crucial roles in providing assistance and emotional
support. Caregivers can share their experiences,
exchange caregiving strategies, and find solace in
knowing that others understand the unique
challenges they face.

7. Building a Sense of Community:
Being part of a support group creates a sense of
community that extends beyond the virtual or

physical meeting space. Members often form lasting bonds and connections, providing ongoing support that transcends the challenges of CAD. This sense of community contributes to a feeling of belonging and reduces the sense of isolation that can accompany chronic health conditions.

8. Advocacy and Awareness:
Support groups often engage in advocacy efforts, raising awareness about CAD and related issues. Members can collectively work towards dispelling misconceptions, promoting heart health initiatives, and advocating for policies that benefit individuals living with CAD.

In conclusion, joining support groups and communities is a transformative experience for individuals affected by CAD. The collective strength, shared knowledge, and emotional support derived from these groups empower individuals to face the challenges of CAD with resilience, fostering a community-driven approach to heart health.

Communicating Effectively with Loved Ones

Effective communication with loved ones is a cornerstone of navigating life with coronary artery disease (CAD). The impact of a CAD diagnosis extends beyond the individual, influencing the dynamics of relationships. Here's a deeper exploration of the nuances involved in communicating effectively with loved ones in the context of CAD.

Communication about CAD should be approached with openness and honesty. Sharing the diagnosis, treatment plan, and potential lifestyle changes is a collaborative process that involves not only providing information but also fostering a space for dialogue. Encouraging loved ones to express their feelings, concerns, and questions creates a two-way channel for understanding and support.

Empathy plays a pivotal role in effective communication. Understanding that a CAD diagnosis can evoke a range of emotions in both the individual and their loved ones, including fear, anxiety, and uncertainty, is crucial. Actively listening to each other's concerns and validating emotions helps build a foundation of trust and support.

It's important to recognize that the impact of CAD extends to daily life and relationships. Communicating about potential adjustments in routines, roles, or expectations is essential. Whether discussing changes in physical activity, dietary habits, or the need for additional support, involving loved ones in these conversations ensures a shared understanding and a collaborative approach to managing CAD.

In moments of frustration or stress, maintaining open lines of communication becomes even more critical. Expressing feelings and concerns as they arise prevents the buildup of tension. Loved ones can offer emotional support, but effective communication allows for the articulation of needs and preferences, ensuring that everyone involved feels heard and understood.

Education is a continuous process in the context of CAD. Loved ones may not initially grasp the complexities of the condition, and ongoing communication helps in providing updates, sharing insights gained from medical appointments, and discussing any changes in the treatment plan. This shared knowledge reinforces a sense of unity in facing the challenges presented by CAD.

Lastly, effective communication involves recognizing that each person may have a unique way of processing information and coping with stress. Some may prefer direct and detailed discussions, while others may need time to absorb information before engaging in conversation. Tailoring communication styles to the individual preferences of loved ones contributes to a more supportive and understanding environment.

In essence, communicating effectively with loved ones about CAD is an ongoing and dynamic process. It requires a blend of openness, empathy, and adaptability. By fostering a space where thoughts and emotions can be shared freely, individuals and their loved ones can navigate the complexities of CAD together, strengthening relationships and creating a supportive network for overall well-being.

Chapter 5: Emotional Well-being

Coping with Anxiety and Depression

Coping with anxiety and depression, especially in the context of coronary artery disease (CAD), demands a thoughtful and compassionate approach. Mental health is intimately intertwined with cardiovascular well-being, and addressing these challenges requires effective communication, understanding, and proactive strategies.

Opening up about feelings of anxiety and depression is a crucial first step. Individuals with CAD often face heightened emotional stress due to concerns about their health, the impact on daily life, and the future. Encouraging open dialogue with loved ones creates an atmosphere where these emotions can be shared without judgment.

Empathy plays a central role in coping with anxiety and depression. Loved ones should strive to understand the unique challenges faced by individuals with CAD, acknowledging the emotional burden that accompanies the condition. Creating a non-judgmental space where feelings are validated fosters a sense of emotional support and reduces the stigma often associated with mental health struggles.

Seeking professional help is an essential component of coping with anxiety and depression. Mental health professionals, such as therapists or counselors, bring specialized expertise to address these challenges. Collaboratively involving loved ones in therapy sessions, when appropriate, can enhance the understanding of coping mechanisms and provide tools for both the individual and their support system.

Encouraging healthy coping mechanisms is vital. This can include mindfulness practices, relaxation techniques, and engaging in activities that bring joy and relaxation. Physical exercise, known for its positive impact on mental health, is particularly beneficial and can be adapted to individual capabilities.

Addressing the potential impact of medications on mental health is another important consideration. Some medications prescribed for CAD may have side effects that influence mood. Open communication with healthcare providers about any changes in mental health allows for adjustments in treatment plans while ensuring comprehensive care.

Understanding that coping with anxiety and depression is an ongoing process is crucial. Individuals with CAD may face fluctuations in their mental health, influenced by various factors such as changes in health status, treatment adjustments, or external stressors. Loved ones should remain vigilant, offer continuous support, and encourage seeking professional help when needed.

In conclusion, coping with anxiety and depression in the context of CAD requires a multifaceted and collaborative approach. Open communication, empathy, seeking professional help, and promoting healthy coping mechanisms create a supportive framework for individuals facing the complex intersection of mental and cardiovascular health. This ongoing process aims to foster resilience, improve overall well-being, and enhance the quality of life for individuals navigating these challenges.

Finding Joy and Purpose in Everyday Life

Finding joy and purpose in everyday life is a transformative endeavor that enriches well-being and brings a sense of fulfillment. Especially for individuals facing challenges like coronary artery disease (CAD), discovering moments of joy and purpose becomes a vital aspect of holistic health.

1. Gratitude Practices:
Cultivating gratitude for the small, positive aspects of daily life can significantly enhance well-being. Taking a moment each day to reflect on what one is grateful for can shift focus towards the positive, fostering a sense of contentment and joy.

2. Mindfulness and Presence:
Embracing mindfulness involves being fully present in the current moment. Whether savoring a cup of tea, enjoying nature, or engaging in daily activities with focused attention, mindfulness encourages a deeper connection with one's surroundings, promoting joy in simple experiences.

3. Pursuing Passions:
Identifying and actively pursuing personal passions brings a profound sense of purpose. Whether it's a hobby, creative endeavor, or learning a new skill, engaging in activities that

resonate with one's interests fosters a sense of accomplishment and joy.

4. Connection with Loved Ones:
Nurturing meaningful relationships contributes to a sense of purpose. Spending quality time with loved ones, sharing experiences, and maintaining connections create a supportive social network that enhances emotional well-being.

5. Acts of Kindness:
Engaging in acts of kindness, no matter how small has a ripple effect on one's sense of purpose and joy. Helping others, expressing kindness, and contributing to the well-being of the community fosters a sense of fulfillment.

6. Embracing Nature:
Connecting with nature has a profound impact on overall well-being. Whether it's a leisurely walk in a park, tending to a garden, or simply appreciating the beauty of the outdoors, nature provides a source of joy and inspiration.

7. Setting Meaningful Goals:
Establishing realistic and meaningful goals, whether short-term or long-term, instills a sense of purpose. Goals provide direction, motivation, and a sense of accomplishment when achieved, contributing to an overall positive outlook on life.

8. Mind-Body Practices:
Engaging in mind-body practices such as yoga, tai
chi, or meditation promotes a holistic sense of
well-being. These practices not only enhance
physical health but also contribute to mental
clarity, emotional balance, and a deeper connection
with oneself.

9. Learning and Growth:
Continual learning and personal growth contribute
to a sense of purpose. Whether through formal
education, reading, or acquiring new skills, the
pursuit of knowledge instills a sense of curiosity
and enthusiasm for life.

10. Reflecting on Values:
Taking time to reflect on personal values and
aligning daily activities with these values provides
a compass for living a purpose-driven life.
Understanding what matters most helps guide
choices and actions toward a more fulfilling
existence.

In essence, finding joy and purpose in everyday
life involves a mindful and intentional approach.
It's about appreciating the present moment,
nurturing connections, pursuing passions, and
aligning daily choices with one's values. For
individuals navigating health challenges like CAD,
this pursuit becomes even more significant,

contributing to a holistic and enriched quality of
life.

The Importance Of A Positive Mindset

A positive mindset holds profound importance in
shaping one's overall well-being and navigating
life's challenges, including those associated with
coronary artery disease (CAD). It goes beyond
mere optimism; it encompasses an adaptive and
resilient approach to circumstances, fostering
emotional strength, physical health, and a higher
quality of life.

Maintaining a positive mindset is instrumental in
managing stress. Individuals with a positive
outlook are better equipped to cope with the
emotional impact of health challenges, reducing
the physiological stress response. This, in turn,
contributes to better cardiovascular health and an
enhanced ability to handle the complexities of
CAD.

A positive mindset also plays a pivotal role in the
healing process. Studies have shown that

individuals with a positive attitude toward their recovery tend to experience better outcomes. The mind-body connection is powerful, and a constructive mindset can positively influence the body's response to treatment, potentially expediting recovery.

Moreover, a positive outlook fosters resilience in the face of setbacks. Living with CAD may involve lifestyle changes, medical interventions, and occasional challenges. A positive mindset helps individuals adapt to these changes, view setbacks as opportunities for growth, and persist in their efforts to manage the condition effectively.

In the context of CAD, where stress and anxiety can exacerbate symptoms, cultivating a positive mindset contributes to better mental health. It involves reframing negative thoughts, focusing on strengths, and embracing a hopeful perspective. This mental resilience not only enhances emotional well-being but also positively impacts physical health, potentially influencing factors like blood pressure and immune function.

Social connections are a significant aspect of health, and a positive mindset facilitates meaningful relationships. Individuals who approach interactions with optimism tend to create a supportive environment, attracting positive energy and fostering connections that contribute to emotional well-being.

Ultimately, the importance of a positive mindset lies in its transformative effect on the overall human experience. It influences how individuals perceive challenges, approach relationships, and engage with life. For those facing the complexities of CAD, a positive mindset becomes a powerful ally, shaping not only the journey of managing the condition but also the broader narrative of a fulfilling and resilient life.

Chapter 6: Creating a Heart-Healthy Environment

Designing Your Living Space for Cardiovascular Wellness

Designing your living space with cardiovascular wellness in mind is a holistic approach that integrates elements to promote physical health, reduce stress, and create an environment conducive to well-being. Consideration of both the physical and emotional aspects of your living space contributes to a heart-healthy lifestyle.

1. Physical Activity Integration:
Incorporate spaces for physical activity within your home. Designate areas for exercises such as yoga, stretching, or light cardio workouts. This encourages regular movement, contributing to cardiovascular fitness. Ensure sufficient natural light in these spaces to boost mood and energy levels.

2. Heart-Healthy Kitchen Design:
Design your kitchen with heart-healthy eating in
mind. Ensure easy access to fresh fruits,
vegetables, and other heart-healthy foods.
Organize the kitchen to facilitate efficient meal
preparation, promoting a balanced and nutritious
diet crucial for cardiovascular wellness.

3. Stress-Reducing Colors and Décor:
Choose calming colors and décor that reduce
stress. Soft blues, greens, and neutral tones can
create a soothing atmosphere. Incorporate elements
like indoor plants or artwork that evoke positive
emotions and contribute to a sense of tranquility.

4. Natural Light and Ventilation:
Maximize natural light and ventilation in your
living space. Exposure to natural light has been
linked to improved mood and overall well-being.
Adequate ventilation supports respiratory health
and creates a fresh and invigorating environment.

5. Comfortable and Ergonomic Furniture:
Select comfortable and ergonomic furniture that
supports good posture and encourages movement.
Properly designed furniture contributes to overall
physical well-being, reducing the risk of
musculoskeletal issues and promoting an active
lifestyle.

6. Declutter for Mental Clarity:

Maintain an organized and clutter-free living space. Clutter can contribute to stress and anxiety, affecting mental well-being. Creating a clean and organized environment supports mental clarity and contributes to a more relaxed atmosphere.

7. Restful Bedroom Environment:
Design your bedroom to promote restful sleep, a crucial component of cardiovascular health. Choose a comfortable mattress and pillows, use blackout curtains to control light, and keep the room cool and quiet for optimal sleep quality.

8. Relaxation Zones:
Designate areas for relaxation and stress reduction. Whether it's a cozy reading nook, a meditation corner, or a comfortable lounge area, having dedicated spaces for relaxation contributes to overall mental and emotional well-being.

9. Heart-Healthy Art and Inspirational Elements:
Incorporate art and elements that inspire and uplift. Consider artwork depicting nature scenes, motivational quotes, or personal mementos that evoke positive emotions. Surrounding yourself with uplifting elements contributes to a positive mindset.

10. Greenery and Nature Integration:
Integrate greenery and natural elements into your living space. Plants not only improve air quality

but also have a calming effect. Create a connection with nature by strategically placing indoor plants or incorporating natural materials in your décor.

In conclusion, designing your living space for cardiovascular wellness involves a thoughtful combination of physical and emotional considerations. By integrating elements that support physical activity, heart-healthy eating, stress reduction, and overall well-being, you create an environment that positively influences your cardiovascular health and enhances your quality of life.

Workplace Strategies for CAD Patients

Implementing workplace strategies for individuals with coronary artery disease (CAD) is essential to support their well-being and ensure a conducive and manageable work environment. These strategies focus on accommodating health needs, managing stress, and fostering a supportive workplace culture.

1. Flexible Work Arrangements:
Consider offering flexible work hours or remote work options. This provides individuals with CAD the flexibility to manage medical appointments, adhere to treatment plans, and address fatigue or

symptom flare-ups without compromising their professional responsibilities.

2. Ergonomic Workstations:
Design workstations with ergonomic principles to support physical health. Ensure proper chair and desk heights, encourage good posture, and provide equipment that reduces strain. This can contribute to overall comfort and minimize physical stress.

3. Breaks and Movement Opportunities:
Encourage regular breaks and movement opportunities during the workday. Individuals with CAD benefit from incorporating short walks or stretching exercises to promote circulation and reduce sedentary behavior. Design break areas that facilitate relaxation.

4. Stress Management Programs:
Implement stress management programs within the workplace. This can include workshops, mindfulness sessions, or access to resources that help employees manage stress effectively. Reducing workplace stress is crucial for individuals with CAD, as stress can impact cardiovascular health.

5. Health and Wellness Initiatives:
Promote health and wellness initiatives that encourage a heart-healthy lifestyle. This could involve providing nutritious snacks, organizing

fitness challenges, or offering resources on maintaining a healthy diet. Supportive workplace environments foster overall well-being.

6. Clear Communication Channels:
Establish clear communication channels between employees and management. This allows individuals with CAD to express their needs, discuss accommodations, and address concerns openly. Open communication contributes to a more supportive and understanding workplace culture.

7. Designated Rest Areas:
Provide designated rest areas where employees can take a break and relax. For individuals with CAD, having a quiet space for rest or meditation can be beneficial, especially during times of heightened stress or when managing symptoms.

8. Emergency Response Plans:
Ensure that emergency response plans consider the needs of employees with CAD. This may involve training staff on responding to medical emergencies, having accessible defibrillators, and creating a workplace environment that prioritizes health and safety.

9. Encourage Regular Health Checkups:
Promote a workplace culture that encourages regular health checkups. Offer flexibility for

employees to attend medical appointments without fear of repercussions. Regular checkups are essential for monitoring and managing CAD effectively.

10. Sensitivity Training:
Conduct sensitivity training to raise awareness about CAD and other cardiovascular conditions. This can help colleagues and supervisors better understand the challenges faced by individuals with CAD, fostering a more inclusive and empathetic workplace culture.

By implementing these workplace strategies, employers can create an environment that not only accommodates the needs of individuals with CAD but also promotes a culture of well-being and support. Recognizing the importance of health, both physical and mental, contributes to a workplace that values its employees' overall health and helps them thrive in their professional roles.

Travel Tips for Individuals with Heart Conditions

Traveling with a heart condition, such as coronary artery disease (CAD), requires careful planning and consideration of health needs. Here are some travel tips for individuals with heart conditions to ensure a safe and enjoyable journey:

1. Consult Your Healthcare Provider:
Before planning any trip, consult with your healthcare provider. Discuss your travel plans, ensure that your health is stable for travel, and obtain any necessary medical advice or documentation.

2. Carry Essential Medications:
Ensure you have an adequate supply of your medications for the entire duration of your trip. Pack medications in their original containers, and bring a list of medications, dosages, and your doctor's contact information.

3. Create a Health Information Card:
Carry a card with essential health information, including your medical history, allergies, current medications, and emergency contacts. Keep this card in your wallet or travel documents for quick reference.

4. Plan for Medication Time Zones:
If you're crossing time zones, work with your healthcare provider to establish a medication schedule that aligns with your destination. This helps maintain consistent control of your condition.

5. Stay Hydrated:
Proper hydration is crucial for cardiovascular health. Carry a reusable water bottle and stay hydrated, especially during air travel where cabin air can be dehydrating.

6. Choose Destinations Wisely:
Consider destinations that align with your health needs. High-altitude locations or extreme climates may impact individuals with heart conditions, so choose destinations that pose minimal risks.

7. Inform Travel Companions:
Make sure your travel companions are aware of your heart condition, know how to assist in case of an emergency, and are familiar with the location of your medications.

8. Pack a Basic First Aid Kit:
Include a basic first aid kit with items like bandages, pain relievers, and any specific medications or medical supplies recommended by your healthcare provider.

9. Know the Location of Medical Facilities:
Research and note the locations of medical facilities, hospitals, and pharmacies at your travel destination. This information can be crucial in case of unexpected health issues.

10. Plan for Rest:
Consider your energy levels and plan for rest periods during your trip. Avoid overexertion, especially in unfamiliar environments, and listen to your body's signals.

11. Inform Transportation Providers:
If using public transportation, inform airlines, bus companies, or cruise lines about your condition. Some may provide additional assistance or accommodations if needed.

12. Wear a Medical Alert Bracelet:
Consider wearing a medical alert bracelet that indicates your heart condition. This can provide crucial information in case of an emergency, even if you are unable to communicate.

13. Travel Insurance:
Invest in travel insurance that covers potential health-related issues. Ensure that your policy covers pre-existing conditions and provides adequate medical coverage.

Remember that every individual's health needs are unique, so tailor these tips based on your specific condition and requirements. By taking proactive measures and planning, individuals with heart conditions can enjoy safe and fulfilling travel experiences.

Chapter 7: Holistic Approaches to Heart Health

Integrating Complementary Therapies

Integrating complementary therapies into conventional healthcare represents a holistic approach to promoting well-being and managing various health conditions, including coronary artery disease (CAD). Complementary therapies, often used alongside standard medical treatments, encompass a range of practices and modalities that address the physical, emotional, and spiritual aspects of an individual's health.

One of the key aspects of integrating complementary therapies into CAD management is the recognition of the interconnectedness of mind and body. Conventional treatments for CAD primarily focus on the physical aspects, such as medication and surgical interventions. However, complementary therapies take a broader view, acknowledging the impact of mental and emotional well-being on cardiovascular health.

Mind-body practices, including meditation, yoga, and deep-breathing exercises, have gained recognition for their positive effects on cardiovascular health. These practices not only promote relaxation and stress reduction but also have been associated with improvements in blood pressure, heart rate variability, and overall heart function. Integrating such practices into CAD management recognizes the importance of addressing both the physiological and psychological aspects of the condition.

Acupuncture, an ancient Chinese practice, is another complementary therapy that has shown promise in cardiovascular health. Studies suggest that acupuncture may help in lowering blood pressure and reducing inflammation, contributing to the overall management of CAD. While it is not a replacement for standard medical treatments, acupuncture exemplifies the collaborative and integrative nature of combining conventional and complementary approaches.

Dietary and nutritional interventions are integral components of CAD management, and certain complementary therapies focus on optimizing nutritional choices. Herbal supplements, such as garlic or omega-3 fatty acids, have been explored for their potential cardiovascular benefits. Integrating these supplements under the guidance of healthcare professionals allows for a comprehensive approach to nutrition, complementing standard dietary recommendations.

Massage therapy, often regarded as a relaxation technique, can contribute to stress reduction and improved circulation. While it may not directly treat CAD, incorporating massage into a holistic care plan can enhance overall well-being and support cardiovascular health indirectly by promoting relaxation and reducing tension.

Furthermore, integrative healthcare models often involve collaboration between conventional healthcare providers and practitioners of complementary therapies. This interdisciplinary approach allows for comprehensive care, with healthcare professionals working together to address the diverse needs of individuals with CAD.

It's crucial to emphasize that the integration of complementary therapies into CAD management should be approached with careful consideration and under the guidance of qualified healthcare professionals. Communication between patients and their healthcare team is paramount to ensure that complementary therapies align with the overall treatment plan and do not interfere with prescribed medications or interventions.

In conclusion, the integration of complementary therapies into CAD management signifies a shift toward a more patient-centered and holistic approach to health. By recognizing and addressing the multifaceted aspects of well-being, individuals with CAD can benefit from a comprehensive care plan that combines the strengths of conventional medicine and complementary therapies, ultimately promoting a more balanced and resilient approach to cardiovascular health.

Mindfulness and meditation techniques

Mindfulness and meditation techniques are powerful practices that promote mental clarity, emotional well-being, and overall stress reduction. Rooted in ancient contemplative traditions, these techniques have gained widespread recognition for their positive impact on various aspects of health, including cardiovascular well-being. Here, we explore some mindfulness and meditation techniques that individuals, including those with coronary artery disease (CAD), can incorporate into their daily lives.

1. Mindful Breathing (Mindful Awareness):
Mindful breathing involves paying attention to the breath as it naturally flows in and out. Sit or lie comfortably, focus your attention on your breath, and observe each inhalation and exhalation. This technique promotes a sense of calm and helps anchor the mind to the present moment.

2. Loving-Kindness Meditation:
Loving-kindness meditation, or Metta meditation, involves directing positive thoughts and feelings towards oneself and others. Start by generating feelings of love and compassion for yourself, then extend these feelings to loved ones, acquaintances, and even those you may have challenges with. This practice fosters a sense of connection and goodwill.

3. Body Scan Meditation:
In a body scan meditation, bring attention to different parts of the body systematically. Start from your toes and gradually move upward, noticing any sensations, tensions, or areas of relaxation. This practice enhances body awareness and can be particularly beneficial for releasing physical tension.

4. Guided Meditation:

Guided meditations involve following the instructions of a teacher or recording. This can be particularly helpful for beginners. Guided sessions often focus on relaxation, mindfulness, or specific intentions, providing a structured approach to meditation.

5. Mindful Walking:
Mindful walking involves paying full attention to the act of walking. Feel the sensation of each step, notice the movements of your body, and be present in the experience. This practice can be done indoors or outdoors and offers a way to incorporate mindfulness into daily activities.

6. Mindful Eating:
Mindful eating involves savoring each bite of food with full attention. Pay attention to the flavors, textures, and sensations as you eat. This practice not only promotes healthier eating habits but also fosters a deeper connection with the act of nourishing your body.

7. Transcendental Meditation (TM):
Transcendental Meditation is a specific form of mantra meditation. Practitioners repeat a mantra silently, allowing the mind to settle into a state of deep restful awareness. TM has been studied for its positive effects on stress reduction and overall well-being.

8. Breath Awareness Meditation:
Similar to mindful breathing, breath awareness
meditation involves gently bringing attention to the
breath. Focus on the sensation of breathing,
whether it's the rise and fall of the chest or the flow
of air through the nostrils. This technique enhances
concentration and promotes relaxation.

9. Mindful Yoga:
Mindful yoga combines physical postures with
breath awareness and meditation. It emphasizes the
integration of movement and mindfulness,
fostering flexibility, balance, and a sense of calm.
Yoga can be adapted to various skill levels and
physical abilities.

10. Progressive Muscle Relaxation:
This technique involves systematically tensing and
then relaxing different muscle groups. Start with
the toes and work your way up to the head,
releasing tension throughout the body. Progressive
muscle relaxation is effective in promoting
physical and mental relaxation.

Incorporating mindfulness and meditation into
daily life can contribute to a sense of balance and
well-being. Individuals, including those managing
CAD, can explore these techniques to discover
which resonates most with their preferences and
needs. It's essential to approach these practices

with an open mind, recognizing that consistency over time often yields the most significant benefits.

Exploring Alternative Healing Practices

Exploring alternative healing practices opens the door to a diverse realm of therapeutic approaches that extend beyond conventional medicine. Embraced for centuries across cultures, these practices offer unique perspectives on well-being, focusing on the interconnectedness of mind, body, and spirit. While alternative healing does not replace traditional medical interventions, it provides individuals, including those with conditions like coronary artery disease (CAD), with additional tools to enhance overall health.

One notable facet of alternative healing is acupuncture, rooted in traditional Chinese medicine. Acupuncture involves the insertion of thin needles into specific points on the body, aiming to balance the flow of vital energy, or qi. Some individuals with CAD find relief in acupuncture for managing symptoms like stress and hypertension, showcasing the potential synergy between ancient practices and modern health needs.

Herbal medicine is another alternative approach that draws on the healing properties of plants. Herbal remedies, whether in the form of teas, tinctures, or supplements, have been used to address various health concerns. While caution is necessary to ensure compatibility with prescribed medications, some herbs are explored for their potential cardiovascular benefits, such as garlic for its reported impact on cholesterol levels.

Energy-based therapies, like Reiki and Healing Touch, operate on the principle that the body has subtle energy fields that can be influenced to promote healing. Practitioners use their hands to channel energy into the body, fostering relaxation and balance. Although the mechanisms behind these therapies may be less understood, some individuals report improved well-being and stress reduction.

Mind-body practices, such as tai chi and qigong, combine movement, breath, and meditation to promote balance and harmony. These ancient Chinese practices are known for enhancing physical and mental well-being, making them valuable components of a holistic approach to health.

Holistic approaches like Ayurveda, originating from ancient Indian traditions, emphasize individualized wellness plans based on one's unique constitution or dosha. Dietary recommendations, lifestyle adjustments, and herbal remedies are tailored to support overall balance, considering the interconnected nature of body and mind.

The exploration of alternative healing practices also encompasses mind-focused techniques like hypnotherapy and biofeedback. These approaches leverage the power of the mind to influence physical responses, offering potential benefits for stress reduction, pain management, and overall mental well-being.

It's essential to approach alternative healing practices with an informed and discerning mindset. While some individuals find profound benefits, others may not experience the same effects. Collaboration with healthcare professionals is crucial to ensure that alternative practices align with individual health needs, complementing rather than conflicting with conventional treatments.

Chapter 8: Navigating

Challenges and Setbacks

Coping with Flare-Ups and Complications
Coping with flare-ups and complications is an inherent challenge for individuals managing chronic health conditions, such as coronary artery disease (CAD). Despite diligent management and adherence to treatment plans, there may be instances when symptoms intensify or unexpected complications arise. Navigating these moments requires resilience, proactive communication with healthcare providers, and a personalized approach to self-care.

Flare-ups in CAD, often characterized by an exacerbation of symptoms like chest pain or shortness of breath, can be disconcerting. The first step in coping is to recognize and acknowledge these changes in health status. Ignoring or downplaying symptoms may delay necessary interventions. Swift communication with healthcare providers is paramount, allowing for timely adjustments to medications or treatment plans.

A proactive role in self-care becomes crucial during flare-ups. This includes adhering strictly to prescribed medications, adopting lifestyle modifications, and prioritizing rest. Understanding personal triggers for flare-ups, whether related to stress, dietary choices, or physical activity, empowers individuals to make informed decisions that mitigate exacerbations.

Complications, such as adverse reactions to medications or unexpected medical events, can introduce additional layers of stress. In these situations, clear communication with healthcare providers is imperative. Prompt reporting of symptoms or concerns enables healthcare professionals to assess the situation comprehensively and make necessary adjustments to the treatment plan.

Emotional well-being is an integral aspect of coping with flare-ups and complications. The anxiety and uncertainty that accompany health setbacks can contribute to emotional distress. Engaging in mindfulness and stress-reduction practices, such as meditation or deep breathing exercises, can provide a sense of calm and support mental resilience during challenging times.

Support systems play a crucial role in navigating flare-ups and complications. Communicating openly with family, friends, or support groups fosters understanding and provides an emotional anchor. Sharing experiences and seeking advice from those who have faced similar challenges can offer practical insights and a sense of camaraderie.

Moreover, healthcare providers can guide individuals through coping strategies tailored to their specific health needs. Education on recognizing early warning signs, creating an emergency action plan, and understanding when to seek immediate medical attention empowers individuals to actively participate in their care.

Overcoming psychological hurdles

Overcoming psychological hurdles is a crucial aspect of managing and adapting to life with coronary artery disease (CAD). The psychological impact of a chronic health condition can manifest in various ways, including stress, anxiety, depression, and fear. Addressing these psychological hurdles is essential for promoting mental well-being and enhancing overall quality of life.

One of the primary psychological hurdles individuals with CAD may face is the fear of the unknown. A CAD diagnosis can bring uncertainties about the future, treatment outcomes, and lifestyle changes. Overcoming this hurdle involves gaining knowledge and understanding the condition. Education about CAD, its management, and lifestyle modifications empowers individuals to make informed decisions, fostering a sense of control and reducing anxiety.

Another common psychological challenge is adapting to lifestyle changes. CAD often necessitates adjustments in diet, physical activity, and overall daily routines. The process of adapting to these changes can be emotionally taxing. Creating a gradual and realistic plan, seeking support from healthcare providers, and involving loved ones in the process can ease the psychological burden associated with lifestyle modifications.

Stress management is paramount in overcoming psychological hurdles related to CAD. Chronic stress can exacerbate cardiovascular symptoms and impact overall health. Implementing stress-reduction techniques, such as mindfulness, meditation, or engaging in relaxing activities, provides individuals with practical tools to navigate the emotional challenges associated with CAD.

Addressing the psychological impact of CAD also involves acknowledging and managing feelings of sadness or depression. Chronic health conditions can influence emotional well-being, and seeking professional support, such as therapy or counseling, can be instrumental in coping with these feelings. Open communication with healthcare providers about emotional struggles ensures a comprehensive approach to care.

Moreover, overcoming psychological hurdles often requires reframing negative thought patterns. Shifting focus from limitations to possibilities, recognizing personal strengths, and celebrating small victories contribute to a positive mindset. Building resilience involves cultivating a mindset that views challenges as opportunities for growth rather than insurmountable obstacles.

Social support plays a crucial role in overcoming psychological hurdles. Connecting with loved ones, sharing experiences with individuals facing similar challenges, and participating in support groups foster a sense of community. Social connections provide emotional support, reduce feelings of isolation, and contribute to a more optimistic outlook.

Overcoming psychological hurdles associated with CAD is a dynamic and multifaceted process. It involves gaining knowledge, adapting to lifestyle changes, managing stress, addressing emotional well-being, and fostering social connections. By actively engaging with these aspects, individuals can navigate the psychological challenges of CAD with resilience, promoting a holistic approach to their overall health and well-being.

Seeking Professional Help When Needed

Seeking professional help when needed is a vital aspect of managing various challenges in life, including those related to health, relationships, and emotional well-being. For individuals navigating conditions like coronary artery disease (CAD), recognizing when to seek professional assistance is a proactive step toward comprehensive care and improved overall quality of life.

One of the primary reasons to seek professional help when dealing with CAD is to address emotional well-being. The psychological impact of a chronic health condition can be profound, leading to feelings of stress, anxiety, or depression. Mental health professionals, such as therapists or counselors, are equipped to provide support, coping strategies, and a safe space for individuals to express and navigate their emotions effectively.

Moreover, seeking professional help becomes crucial when managing the complexities of treatment plans and lifestyle adjustments. Healthcare providers, including cardiologists, nutritionists, and rehabilitation specialists, play integral roles in guiding individuals with CAD. Regular check-ups, consultations, and collaboration with healthcare professionals ensure that treatment plans are tailored to individual needs, and any adjustments can be made promptly based on evolving health conditions.

Individuals facing CAD may also benefit from seeking professional assistance for lifestyle modifications. Dietitians can provide guidance on heart-healthy nutrition, helping individuals make informed choices that support cardiovascular health. Exercise physiologists or physical therapists can create personalized fitness plans, considering individual capabilities and restrictions.

Furthermore, professional help is essential for managing medications effectively. Cardiologists and pharmacists play key roles in prescribing and adjusting medications, monitoring potential side effects, and ensuring optimal adherence to the prescribed regimen. This collaborative approach helps maintain cardiovascular health and reduces the risk of complications.

When facing challenges in interpersonal relationships or struggling with the emotional impact of CAD on family dynamics, couples or family therapy can be beneficial. These therapeutic approaches provide a platform for open communication, understanding, and collaborative problem-solving, fostering a supportive environment for both individuals with CAD and their loved ones.

Recognizing the need for professional help is a sign of strength and proactive self-care. It acknowledges that managing CAD is a collaborative effort that extends beyond individual capabilities. Seeking professional assistance when needed reflects a commitment to overall well-being and a willingness to address the multifaceted aspects of living with a chronic health condition.

Chapter 9: Planning for the Future

Long-Term Management Strategies

Long-term management strategies for coronary artery disease (CAD) are crucial for sustaining cardiovascular health, preventing complications, and enhancing overall well-being. These strategies encompass a multifaceted approach, combining lifestyle modifications, medication adherence, regular medical monitoring, and a proactive mindset. Here are key elements of effective long-term management for CAD:

1. Adherence to Medications:
Consistent adherence to prescribed medications is paramount for managing CAD. Medications such as antiplatelets, beta-blockers, statins, and angiotensin-converting enzyme (ACE) inhibitors play critical roles in controlling symptoms, preventing complications, and improving overall cardiovascular outcomes. Regular communication

with healthcare providers is essential to address any concerns or potential side effects.

2. Heart-Healthy Lifestyle:
Adopting and maintaining a heart-healthy lifestyle is foundational for long-term CAD management. This includes:

  - Balanced Diet: Emphasize a diet rich in fruits, vegetables, whole grains, lean proteins, and low-fat dairy. Limit saturated and trans fats, cholesterol, sodium, and added sugars.

  - Regular Physical Activity: Engage in regular aerobic exercise, such as brisk walking, cycling, or swimming. Aim for at least 150 minutes of moderate-intensity exercise per week, as recommended by health guidelines.

  - Tobacco Cessation: Quitting smoking is crucial for cardiovascular health. Smoking cessation programs and support can significantly improve long-term outcomes.

  - Moderate Alcohol Consumption: If alcohol is consumed, do so in moderation. For men, this typically means up to two drinks per day, and for women, up to one drink per day.

3. Weight Management:

Maintaining a healthy weight contributes to overall cardiovascular health. Weight management involves a combination of a nutritious diet, regular physical activity, and lifestyle modifications. Achieving and maintaining a healthy weight can positively impact blood pressure, cholesterol levels, and overall heart function.

4. Regular Medical Check-Ups:
Scheduled medical check-ups with healthcare providers are essential for ongoing CAD management. Regular monitoring allows for the assessment of cardiovascular health, adjustment of treatment plans as needed, and early detection of any emerging issues. Blood pressure checks, cholesterol level assessments, and routine screenings contribute to proactive health management.

5. Stress Reduction and Mental Well-Being:
Chronic stress can adversely affect cardiovascular health. Incorporating stress reduction techniques such as mindfulness, meditation, or relaxation exercises is beneficial for long-term CAD management. Additionally, addressing mental well-being through counseling or support groups can provide valuable tools for coping with the emotional aspects of living with a chronic health condition.

6. Diabetes Management:

For individuals with CAD and diabetes, effective management of blood sugar levels is crucial. Regular monitoring, adherence to prescribed medications, and lifestyle modifications are key components of diabetes management that contribute to overall cardiovascular health.

7. Education and Self-Empowerment: Continuous education about CAD and its management empowers individuals to actively participate in their care. Understanding the condition, treatment options, and lifestyle recommendations enables informed decision-making and fosters a proactive mindset in long-term management.

Long-term management of coronary artery disease requires a comprehensive and sustained approach. By integrating these key elements into daily life, individuals can optimize cardiovascular health, minimize complications, and enhance their overall well-being over the course of their journey with CAD.

Financial Planning for Healthcare Costs

Financial planning for healthcare costs is a critical aspect of overall financial well-being, especially for individuals managing chronic conditions like coronary artery disease (CAD). Rising healthcare expenses can have a significant impact on one's financial stability, making proactive planning essential. Here are key strategies for effective financial planning in the context of healthcare costs:

1. Health Insurance Evaluation:
Review and understand your health insurance coverage. Analyze the policy details, including deductibles, copayments, and coverage limits. Consider the specific needs related to CAD, such as medication coverage, cardiac rehabilitation, and specialized treatments. If possible, explore different insurance plans to ensure comprehensive coverage.

2. Emergency Fund:
Establish and maintain an emergency fund specifically earmarked for healthcare expenses. A robust emergency fund can provide a financial buffer in case of unexpected medical costs or emergencies related to CAD. Aim to set aside three to six months' worth of living expenses in this fund.

3. Budgeting for Healthcare:
Incorporate healthcare costs into your budget. Allocate funds for insurance premiums, copayments, prescriptions, and any anticipated

medical expenses related to CAD. Tracking and planning for these costs in advance help avoid financial strain when medical bills arise.

4. Health Savings Account (HSA) or Flexible Spending Account (FSA):
If eligible, contribute to an HSA or FSA. These accounts offer tax advantages and allow you to set aside pre-tax dollars for qualified medical expenses. HSAs, in particular, can also serve as long-term savings for healthcare costs in retirement.

5. Understand Medication Costs:
Be aware of the costs associated with prescribed medications for CAD. Explore generic alternatives or patient assistance programs that may help reduce the financial burden. Regularly review your medication plan with healthcare providers to ensure cost-effective and appropriate options.

6. Negotiate Medical Bills:
If faced with high medical bills, don't hesitate to negotiate with healthcare providers. Many providers are willing to work out payment plans or offer discounts for prompt payment. Discussing your situation and exploring options can potentially reduce the financial impact.

7. Financial Counseling:

Some healthcare facilities provide financial counseling services. If you anticipate significant medical expenses related to CAD, consider seeking guidance from financial counselors. They can help you navigate payment options, understand bills, and explore available assistance programs.

8. Long-Term Care Planning:
Considering potential long-term care needs is part of comprehensive financial planning. Evaluate options for long-term care insurance or explore strategies for covering potential caregiving expenses associated with CAD.

9. Continuously Review and Adjust:
Regularly review your financial plan in light of changing healthcare needs, insurance coverage, and overall financial circumstances. Adjust your budget and savings strategies accordingly to ensure ongoing financial preparedness.

10. Seek Professional Financial Advice:
Consulting with a financial advisor can provide personalized guidance tailored to your specific situation. A financial professional can help you navigate investment strategies, retirement planning, and overall financial goals, taking into account the potential impact of CAD on your financial outlook.

In conclusion, strategic financial planning for healthcare costs is an integral component of overall financial well-being, particularly for individuals managing chronic conditions. By proactively addressing healthcare expenses through insurance evaluation, budgeting, savings, and strategic planning, individuals can better navigate the financial aspects associated with conditions like coronary artery disease.

Advanced Directives and End-of-Life Decisions

Advanced directives and end-of-life decisions are integral components of healthcare planning that empower individuals to communicate their preferences and maintain control over their medical care, especially in critical situations. As medical technology advances and life-prolonging interventions become more complex, the importance of these directives becomes increasingly evident. This essay explores the significance of advanced directives, the ethical considerations surrounding end-of-life decisions, and the impact these choices have on patients, families, and healthcare professionals.

Advanced Directives: Empowering Personal Choices

Advanced directives are legal documents that allow individuals to outline their healthcare preferences in the event they are unable to communicate or make decisions. These directives include components such as living wills, durable power of attorney for healthcare, and do-not-resuscitate (DNR) orders. Living wills express preferences regarding specific medical interventions, while durable power of attorney designates a trusted person to make healthcare decisions on behalf of the individual.

The empowerment derived from advanced directives lies in the ability to articulate personal values, beliefs, and treatment preferences. This proactive approach not only provides clarity for medical professionals but also alleviates the burden on family members who might otherwise grapple with difficult decisions during times of crisis.

Ethical Considerations in End-of-Life Decisions

End-of-life decisions raise ethical considerations that healthcare professionals, patients, and families must navigate delicately. Balancing respect for patient autonomy with beneficence and non-maleficence poses challenges. The principle of autonomy emphasizes an individual's right to make decisions about their own life, even if those decisions involve refusing life-sustaining treatments. However, healthcare professionals also face the ethical obligation to promote the well-being of their patients.

The ethical landscape further evolves when considering cultural, religious, and familial perspectives on end-of-life care. Understanding and respecting diverse beliefs and values is crucial in ensuring that end-of-life decisions align with the individual's cultural and spiritual context.

Impact on Patients, Families, and Healthcare Professionals

For patients, having advanced directives in place fosters a sense of control and peace of mind. It enables them to make decisions consistent with their values, ensuring that medical interventions align with their preferences for quality of life.

Families, often burdened with emotional distress, benefit from the clarity provided by advanced directives. Instead of grappling with uncertainty, they can honor their loved one's wishes and focus on providing emotional support during difficult times.

Healthcare professionals navigate the ethical complexities of end-of-life decisions while striving to uphold patient autonomy and provide compassionate care. Having clear directives helps them navigate treatment plans in alignment with the patient's wishes, reducing moral distress and fostering ethical decision-making.

The Role of Communication and Education

Effective communication is central to the success of advanced directives. Healthcare professionals must engage in open and honest conversations with patients about their values, goals, and fears related to end-of-life care. This communication should extend to family members, ensuring everyone involved is well-informed and supportive of the patient's decisions.

Education plays a pivotal role in increasing awareness and encouraging individuals to create advanced directives. Public campaigns, healthcare seminars, and discussions within communities contribute to a cultural shift where individuals see advanced directives as a responsible and compassionate aspect of their overall healthcare plan.

Conclusion

Advanced directives and end-of-life decisions are cornerstones of patient-centered care and ethical healthcare practices. By empowering individuals to express their preferences and providing a framework for decision-making, advanced directives contribute to a more compassionate, dignified, and patient-focused approach to end-of-life care. As society continues to grapple with the complexities of medical advancements and ethical considerations, fostering open communication and promoting education on advanced directives become crucial steps toward honoring individual autonomy and ensuring dignified end-of-life experiences.

Chapter 10: Inspiring Stories of Resilience

Real-life Experiences of Individuals Thriving with CAD

Real-life experiences of individuals thriving with coronary artery disease (CAD) offer inspiration and insights into the resilience, lifestyle changes, and positive mindset that contribute to a fulfilling life despite the challenges posed by this condition. Here are a few narratives showcasing how individuals have navigated and thrived with CAD:

1. John's Journey to Heart-Healthy Living:
John, diagnosed with CAD in his early 50s, transformed his lifestyle to prioritize heart health. He embraced a balanced diet, rich in fruits, vegetables, and whole grains. Regular exercise became a cornerstone of his routine, with daily walks and supervised cardiac rehabilitation sessions. John's commitment to stress management through meditation and mindfulness played a crucial role in his overall well-being. Today, in his 60s, John not only manages CAD effectively but

has also become an advocate for heart-healthy living in his community.

2. Maria's Empowerment through Education:
Maria, diagnosed with CAD after a heart attack, embarked on a journey of education and self-empowerment. She attended cardiac rehabilitation programs, participated in support groups, and became well-versed in her treatment plan. By actively engaging in her healthcare decisions, Maria not only managed CAD but also found a renewed sense of control and confidence. Her advocacy for patient education has empowered others in her community facing similar challenges.

3. Tom's Triumph Over Adversity:
Tom, diagnosed with CAD in his 40s, faced a series of setbacks, including multiple surgeries and complications. Despite the physical and emotional toll, Tom remained resilient. He embraced cardiac rehabilitation with determination, gradually rebuilding his strength and endurance. Tom's story highlights the importance of perseverance and the supportive role of healthcare providers in helping individuals overcome the hurdles associated with CAD.

4. Emily's Holistic Approach to Well-Being:
Emily, living with CAD, adopted a holistic approach to well-being. In addition to medical management, she explored complementary

therapies such as yoga and meditation. Emily prioritized mental health by seeking counseling to navigate the emotional impact of CAD. By integrating physical, mental, and emotional aspects of health, Emily not only managed her condition effectively but also found a renewed sense of vitality and purpose.

5. Carlos's Supportive Network:
Carlos, diagnosed with CAD in his 60s, credits his thriving journey to the support of his family and friends. Open communication and shared decision-making within his support network contributed to a positive environment. Carlos actively participated in family activities, fostering a sense of normalcy. His experience underscores the significance of social connections and the role of a supportive network in navigating life with CAD.

These real-life experiences highlight that thriving with CAD involves more than medical management alone. Lifestyle modifications, education, mental health support, and a robust support network contribute to individuals not only managing their condition but also leading fulfilling lives. By sharing these stories, we can inspire others facing similar challenges and promote a more comprehensive understanding of life with coronary artery disease.

Triumphs and Lessons Learned from Real-Life Experiences Thriving with CAD

The narratives of individuals thriving with coronary artery disease (CAD) are filled with triumphs that reflect resilience, commitment to health, and a positive mindset. These stories offer valuable lessons that extend beyond medical management, providing insights into the multifaceted journey of living with CAD.

1. Triumphs in Lifestyle Transformation:
The triumphs of individuals like John showcase the transformative power of lifestyle changes. Embracing a heart-healthy diet, incorporating regular exercise, and prioritizing stress management became pivotal aspects of their triumph over CAD. The lesson learned here is that lifestyle modifications, when approached with commitment and consistency, contribute significantly to overall well-being.

2. Empowerment through Education and Advocacy:

Maria's story emphasizes the triumph of empowerment through education. By actively engaging in her healthcare decisions and becoming an advocate for patient education, Maria not only managed CAD effectively but also found a sense of control over her health. The lesson is clear: knowledge is empowering, and individuals who actively seek information about their condition can navigate the complexities of CAD more effectively.

3. Resilience in the Face of Setbacks:
Tom's triumph over adversity highlights the resilience required in the face of setbacks associated with CAD. Despite multiple surgeries and complications, Tom's determination to participate in cardiac rehabilitation became a beacon of strength. The lesson learned is that resilience, coupled with the support of healthcare providers, plays a crucial role in overcoming the challenges inherent in managing CAD.

4. Holistic Well-Being and Purposeful Living:
Emily's holistic approach to well-being reflects a triumph that extends beyond physical health. By prioritizing mental health through complementary therapies and counseling, Emily not only managed her condition but also discovered renewed vitality and purpose. The lesson here is that addressing the mental and emotional aspects of CAD contributes significantly to a more fulfilling life.

5. The Significance of Support Networks:
Carlos's triumph underscores the significance of
supportive networks in the journey with CAD.
Open communication, shared decision-making,
and active participation in family activities created
a positive environment for Carlos. The lesson is
clear: social connections and a supportive network
play a crucial role in navigating the challenges of
living with CAD.

6. Continuous Learning and Adaptation:
Across these triumphs, a common lesson
emerges—the journey with CAD is dynamic,
requiring continuous learning and adaptation. Each
individual's experience underscores the importance
of staying informed, remaining open to new
approaches, and adapting lifestyle strategies as
needed.

Building a Community of Support: Thriving with Coronary Artery Disease

Thriving with coronary artery disease (CAD) goes
beyond individual efforts—it often involves
building a robust community of support. Real-life

stories showcase triumphs that emerge when individuals, families, healthcare providers, and communities come together. Lifestyle transformations, empowerment through education, resilience in the face of setbacks, holistic well-being, and the significance of support networks are common threads.

These narratives reveal that thriving with CAD is not a solitary journey but a collective effort. Lifestyle changes, exemplified by individuals like John, emphasize the impact of community-wide awareness and education. Empowerment, as seen in Maria's story, underscores the value of healthcare providers collaborating with patients in decision-making.

Resilience, a recurring theme, demonstrates the strength derived from not just individual determination but the encouragement of a supportive community. Holistic well-being, exemplified by Emily, emphasizes that healthcare extends beyond physical health, encompassing mental and emotional aspects.

Finally, the significance of support networks, highlighted by Carlos, is a cornerstone in building a community of encouragement. Open communication, shared decision-making, and active participation create an environment where individuals can thrive despite the challenges posed by CAD.

In summary, building a community of support is pivotal for thriving with CAD. These real-life experiences underscore the collective triumphs and lessons learned, emphasizing that when communities unite, individuals can navigate the complexities of CAD with resilience, knowledge, and a sense of purpose. This collective approach not only enhances individual well-being but also contributes to a broader culture of understanding and support for those facing coronary artery disease.

www.ingramcontent.com/pod-product-compliance
Lightning Source LLC
Chambersburg PA
CBHW050739260726

48661CB00001B/311